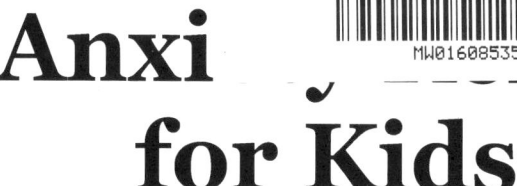

# Anxiety Relief for Kids

*The Complete Workbook to Help Your Child Overcome Worry, Stress, Anger, Depression, Panic Attacks, and Fear (A Parent's Guide with Strategies That Work)*

*By Rachel Stone*

# Table of Contents

**Anxiety Relief for Kids**

Table of Contents

Foreword

Introduction

**Chapter 1: Understanding Child Anxiety**

What Causes Anxiety in Your Child?

**Chapter 2: Anxiety Relief Strategies/Activities Toolbox**

**Chapter 3: Parenting an Anxious Child**

5 Steps to Building a Better Connection with Your Anxious Child

**Chapter 4: Engaging Games and Crafts for Parents and Children**

Apps That Help Your Kids with Anxiety

**Chapter 5: Depression vs. Anger**

What You Can Help Your Child Do to Overcome Depression
How Meditation Will Be Beneficial in Helping Your Child Overcome Anger and Depression

Easy Ways Your Child Can Learn to Meditate
Reassure Your Child to Never Give Up

**Chapter 6: Panic Attacks vs Fear**

The Difference between Panic Attacks and
Fear
What Is Anxiety and Panic Attacks?
Does Your Child Have Anxiety?
Why Is My Child Experiencing Panic Attacks
and Anxiety?
Understanding Anxiety
What Is It Like For Your Child to Live With
Anxiety?
How to Help Your Child Deal and Cope with
Anxiety

**Conclusion**

# Foreword

"My children are the reason I laugh, smile, and get up every morning." - Gena Lee Nolin
This quote represents the feelings of many parents, particularly those who desire the best for their children and family as a whole. This eBook was created for those parents living with children who are suffering from anxiety in the forms of worry, stress, anger, depression, panic attacks, and fear. This workbook is designed to give hope to these parents and let them know that there are practical strategies that can help their child overcome these forms of anxiety.

Harmony within the home is a goal of any good parent and when a child is dealing with fear or stress, this harmony is compromised. This is what makes this book so highly important because it opens the doors of communication between parent and child and puts the power back into the parents' hands. Every good parent dealing with child anxiety issues desires not to feel powerless but instead wants to participate in the child's healing.

The hope of this eBook is to present strategies that are simple to implement and bring harmony back into the home by presenting real solutions that can be utilized in daily life. We will provide proven facts that will bring about real solutions to address each form of anxiety your child may be dealing with. Anxiety disorders are becoming more common as approximately twenty-five percent of all children and teens are now suffering from some form of anxiety and stress-related illness. Allow this book to be your guide to the journey back to your child's healthy and flourishing state of mind.

I wish you the best of luck in implementing these strategies that will bring peace to your child and peace back into your family.

# Introduction

Congratulations on purchasing this book and thank you for doing so.

This eBook will present to you strategies that can be simply implemented to help your child live an anxiety-free life. These signs of anxiety will be addressed by this workbook — worry, stress, anger, depression, panic attacks, and fear. There will be solutions that are not your everyday information presented for each exhibited sign of this stressful condition. When a child is dealing with anxiety, whether out in the open or in secret, it affects the whole family. Signs are exhibited that disrupt the peace of the family dynamics. Often true communication is severed between parent and child because of these anxiety issues. Teens will often attempt to hide these signs and leave parents wondering what is going on with their behavior.

Within these strategies given, parents will be able to communicate better and become an active participant in their child's healing. GAD (General Anxiety Disorders) cause children, especially young teens, to worry daily about everything, no matter how small the issue may be. Children suffering from GAD see everything coming their way as a monumental task to handle. GAD covers a wide range of anxiety symptoms, many of which are addressed in this eBook. This workbook acts as a guide for parents to be able to first identify the disorder and then to choose those strategies that will work to help their child overcome that specific disorder.

The differences, reasons, and triggers will be described for each sign of anxiety to assist the parents in choosing which exercises and strategies will work best for their specific situation. Without a guide for parental assistance, there is little a parent can say or do to stop the incessant worrying that comes with most forms of childhood anxiety. A guide is needed so that the right road to solutions is chosen. The information within this eBook will also be of help to parents on how to personally cope with their child's anxiety disorder. When a parent has no coping skills when it comes to dealing with childhood anxiety, it will only make the situation worse and cause the parent to begin to exhibit signs of their own stress and worry which is counterproductive when it comes to helping their child heal.

This workbook is designed to help parents identify the disorder, target the signs of the specific anxiety disorder, whether worry, stress, fear, etc., and then to choose a practical solution that will work best on a daily basis for their child's specific condition. As the parent, you most likely know your child better than anyone and notice the differences in their behavior. This knowledge will help you to assist your child in healing from their disorder. Utilize this knowledge of your child when deciding which strategy to use and which one will be the most effective.

There are plenty of books on this subject on the market, thanks again for choosing this one! Every effort was made to ensure it is full of as much useful information as possible, please enjoy!

# Chapter 1: Understanding Child Anxiety

Anxiety disorder is one of the most common mental disorders today. It shows itself in many different ways — worry, stress, anger, panic attacks, and constant fear. There are a multitude causes for anxiety. Trauma or unusual amounts of stress are just two reasons why someone would suffer from an anxiety disorder. Anxiety disorders are rising today in children and teens who are exhibiting signs of stress and worry over everyday life situations.

The American Psychiatric Association defines anxiety as "anticipation of a future concern". Our natural fight or flight response to a threatening situation is healthy and can be helpful under normal circumstances, but when we stay in that mode of existence is when the signs of anxiety appear. Often people, children, and adults, who suffer from anxiety disorder are stuck in their concern for the future and feel threatened by everyday issues and remain in the fight or flight state. This is when the natural fight or flight mode becomes dangerous.

The reasons for anxiety disorder vary from person to person — from trauma to being overwhelmed by stressful situations. For kids, these reasons can range from heavy-duty school work to disturbing family situations such as divorce, death, abuse and parental abuse, parent to parent. The reason for the anxiety disorder will determine what the best practical solution is for that specific condition and that particular child. Let's discuss some of the main reasons for childhood anxiety.

Lack of the proper amount of sleep can be a cause for anxiety in children. Simply staying up too late or having loud noises playing, such as music, as well as video games can disrupt a child's sleep pattern. Parents must set proper bedtimes for children and make sure that they will stick to those bedtime rules. Sleep is important for kids, especially when it comes to performance in school. If school performance becomes an issue, that can also exacerbate the anxiety symptoms.

Irrational fears can be a trigger for anxiety symptoms as well. Fear of the unknown, children who must deal with a divorce issue, or any kind of family disturbance. They may see a simple argument as a sign of separation. This is where real communication between parent and child comes into play. It is best for parents not to be in pretend mode, but to be as honest as possible with their children as to what is going on with family situations. The fear of not doing well enough in school because of parental pressure or societal pressure can be another trigger. A child may be actually doing his or her best but may feel inadequate when it comes to perfecting good grades in school. Though their parents may be healthy, many children dwell on the death of their parents, though nothing is significantly wrong. They fear being left alone although there may not be any reason to fear at all. These sorts of irrational fears can bring on anxiety in children that lingers with them from age to age and year to year.

Knowing your child is so important when they are dealing with anxiety issues because the better you actually know your child, the easier it is to determine when their anxiety rises. Parents must pay attention to their child's behavior so that they can notice when behaviors begin to change. Irritability, impatience, insomnia, diving school grades, a lack of being social, and not wanting to be around friends, are all signs that an anxiety attack may be occurring. Constant nervousness, jitteriness, or simply not feeling well, can be signs of upcoming panic attacks. Health is a vital factor when it comes to determining why your child is anxious. A doctor's visit may be necessary to see if there are any physical or biological challenges that may be affecting your child's inability to cope with everyday life.

## Worry

Noticing when your child is overly anxious about something is the job of a vigilant parent who is assisting in ridding that child of anxiety. Constant worrying is a sure sign of anxiety. You may notice that your child is worrying about the near future, asking irrational questions, spending too much time alone as in isolating themselves from family and friends. Communication lines must be open with your child so that you can ask them what or why they are worrying. Sometimes they will know and can express themselves to you, other times they may not know and have a difficult time communicating. This is a sign that there may be some other health issue in the big picture. If they do communicate to you why they are worrying, put their minds at ease about the subject and be open enough for them to speak with you about anything without judgment. This invitation will open the door for clearer and more honest communication. Tell your child when you notice that something is wrong. Don't keep it to yourself.

**Stress**

Stress is one of the main symptoms of anxiety disorders. The simplest thing or task can appear to be something overwhelming. Your child's behavior may seem frantic and erratic, unpredictable. Speak your concerns out loud to your child and tell them that you feel that they are stressed out. Your child may be feeling the stress of obtaining good grades or having the "right" friends in school. They may feel socially inadequate due to peer pressure or teasing in school. Make sure that you listen closely to your child if they choose to tell you what's wrong, and comment gently on their feelings and validate their feelings. Avoid blame and lecturing and allow your child to speak freely and openly without fear of what you may think or feel. Remember this should their time to express themselves, not yours.

## Anger

Anger is a volatile sign of anxiety which many children and young teens experience. Overreacting to situations is a number one sign that anger is a part of your child's anxiety disorder. They may be angry towards you or the family for seemingly no reason at all — but remember to honor their feelings and let them tell you what they feel they are angry about. Do your best as a parent to de-escalate the anger, while still allowing your child to have a voice. You as the parent can set aggression limitations but still let your child know that those feelings of anger are allowed. Notice the warning signs of outbursts and teach your child how to notice those same signs within themselves. Remember, "The truth about rage is that it only dissolves when it is really heard and understood, without reservation." - Carl Rogers

## Depression

Depression — everyone gets the blues sometimes, but childhood depression is a different story. Some people think that childhood is a breeze, the easiest time in one's life. However, this is not true for many children. Another sign of anxiety or even an anxiety trigger is depression in children. Parents should recognize that sadness and depression are two different things. Sadness is often triggered by an event of some kind. It is often a very temporary feeling that is associated with a very specific event. Depression is more like a void of feelings. Your child may go through what appears to be "feeling nothing" about anything. This is a point parents should deeply take notice of — that your child is not responding one way or the other about any situation or circumstance. This is a sign of true depression. Depression is a persistent type of sadness that affects schoolwork, social activities, and family participation.

If you notice a bout of depression in your child, speaking with them about it is the first step. Listening to what they have to say is vitally important and this sign may require a need to see a doctor. With depression symptoms, it is good to know if there is a biological or psychological reason behind it that could call for a need for treatment. Though depression is serious, it can be treated and that treatment depends upon its severity.

## Panic Attacks

Children and teens who suffer from a panic attack disorder often experience bursts of fear and high anxiety moments. These attacks are usually unexpected and startling to the child and the parents. Panic attacks are increased periods of the anxiety disorder that lies beneath it all. So what signs can parents look for when they have children who suffer this disorder? Your child may experience difficulty breathing, irregular heartbeats, dizziness, and lightheadedness. These are the major signs of an upcoming panic attack. Try to keep your child as calm as possible by doing deep breathing exercises. Ask your child if there is anything they want to talk about that may help relieve the attack. If necessary, take your child to a physician to see if there is anything wrong at the moment with their health. Though the symptoms are biological, there may also be extreme stress in your child's life that you are unaware of. This is why noticing the signs become so important so that if your child needs to get something off their chest, they know they can come to you before a full-on panic attack occurs.

## Fear

If your child is experiencing bouts of fear on a constant basis, this can be one of the most disturbing signs of anxiety disorders. Discuss the fearful emotions with your child. Leave room for the emotions to flow and validate these emotions. This is also not a time for judgment but a time for listening to what your child has to say. Some fears may be irrational as we discussed earlier, but your child must be able to express him or herself freely even though you may feel that there is no reason to fear. This is a time when your child's feelings are paramount and they must be honored with gentle and caring conversation. If your child expresses why he or she is afraid, speak with them about the issue and allow them to convey why they have such fear over this particular event or situation. The best action overall, no matter which one or more of these anxiety disorder symptoms your child displays, is to listen and allow them to feel what they are feeling as you help them through this sometimes, debilitating issue.

**Social Anxiety**

Social anxiety is also something that can manifest in a child. Social anxiety disorder is a type of social phobia which is a form of a mental health condition. Social anxiety is described as an excessive fear of social or performance situations and instances, and those who experience social anxiety experience these fears when they are exposed to people with whom they are not familiar with. In children, it may often be mistaken as extreme shyness, and a common behavior pattern here would be your child actively avoiding social situations, even playing with other children.

Children who are socially nervous and anxious will experience feelings of fear, apprehension, and nervousness, often prominent when they think they are going to be in a social situation. They will display this same nervousness and anxiety not just among adults, but other children too. Although the symptoms of social anxiety and shyness are often intertwined with one another, social anxiety is when that fear is taken to a new level. Children who are experiencing social anxiety often try to avoid any form of social interaction because they find it extremely difficult being around people. Social situations become something which is much too stressful for them to handle. Social anxiety can lead to loneliness and isolation because of the constant avoidance of human interaction.

Keep a lookout for the following signs which indicate that your child may be experiencing social anxiety.

- They don't make eye contact.

- They become distressed when they feel they are being teased or criticized.

- They become distressed when they find themselves being in a situation where they are the centre of attention.

- They are visibly distressed, awkward, nervous, and uncomfortable being around new people.

- They become distressed when they feel they are being watched or observed while they are doing something.

- They are easily embarrassed to a point where they start blushing and visibly shaking

# What Causes Anxiety in Your Child?

It is hard to say for sure what causes anxiety. Determining the exact cause is tricky, but research has indicated that it could be caused by a combination of both environmental factors and genetics. Environmental factors here include negative experiences that could leave the individual scarred for life, such as bullying, physical, and/or sexual abuse for example.

**Anxiety Could Be Caused by Genetics**
There is still ongoing research that is attempting to determine just how much genetics play a role in influencing anxiety in a child. Anxiety does appear to be common in families (it runs in the family), but to what extent it is difficult to say for sure. It is still not clear whether anxiety is for certain linked to genetic reasons, or whether it is

something that a child picks up from the adults in the family.

For example, if a parent displays signs of anxiety, the child may learn to develop the same kind of behavior patterns. Children are also susceptible to developing anxiety if they are raised in an environment that is too controlling or overprotective, and this behavior could carry on even until they are adults.

## Anxiety Could Be Caused by the Amygdala

Some experts believe that amygdala, which is a structure in the brain that controls a person's fear response and feelings or thoughts of anxiety, may also be a possible cause for a child's anxiety. This is applicable to both adults and children, as a matter of fact. An overactive amygdala could possibly play a role in the way a person responds to fear, causing them to sometimes react excessively and irrationally which then leads to anxiety. The amygdala is the primary source of where our fear reaction stems from. The amygdala is an important part of the brain in relation to anxiety, especially because it makes you choose between two reactions such as the fight or flight response.

## Anxiety Could Be Caused by the Body's Natural Chemicals

The body's natural chemicals might also have a part to play in the development of anxiety in a child. Serotonin for example, which is a chemical found in the brain, may, in fact, play a key role in this scenario. When the serotonin levels in the brain are not right or imbalanced, it is possible that it could contribute to your child developing anxiety. This is because serotonin is responsible for regulating the mood's that we experience within our bodies.

## Anxiety Could Be Caused By a Past Negative Experience

A past negative experience which caused your child a lot of trauma could also be a reason for their current anxiety now. If they previously experienced fear and humiliation for example, or maybe even some other extreme emotion, they eventually become fearful of experiencing a repeat of this situation. Young children especially who experience bullying, teasing, humiliation, rejection, ridicule, and more, may be more prone to developing anxiety as they progress into adulthood. Naturally, if a situation is going to bring out nothing but feelings of fear, discomfort, anxiety, and sheer panic, all they will want to do is get away from the situation as fast as possible.

# Chapter 2: Anxiety Relief Strategies/Activities Toolbox

Parents play a huge role in how their children handle emotions and feelings they are experiencing. In this chapter, we will discuss some strategies to help your children with anxiety disorders. What roles can you play at home that will help to decrease the amount of worry and stress your child goes through on a daily basis?

**Communication**

Good and clear communication within a family is helpful to a child experiencing anxiety disorder or to keep your children from having this health issue. When a child is unsure of what is going on inside the family dynamics, it can be disturbing and cause worry and fear. Children will begin to make up stories about what is happening when they are unaware of the truth. This is why it is a parent's job to be clear and speak the truth as much as can be understood by the child as often as possible. Because so many marriage issues affect children in a deep way, it is healthy to explain in your child's language what the issues are. Particularly, if there are arguments and tension within the home, it is wise to explain to your child that these arguments or tense discussions are not their fault. You must help to remove the blame that children often undertake when something is going awry within the family unit.

## Question/Answer Sessions

A great idea to assist in the helping of your child's anxiety issues is a question/answer session as often as possible. Sit down with your child in a casual manner or take them to the park or playground and make it a fun session. Ask your child if there is anything on their minds that is causing them to worry about anything. Offer the time and allow your child to ask any question that is on their minds about the family, school, friends, or social issues. This will open your child up to communicating with you on a deeper level. They will begin to feel free to inquire about anything bothering them at the moment. And you will be surprised at what children notice within their home and school environment. They may feel left out in school because they didn't make the cheerleading team, the football team, or drama club. This time set aside for expression and inquiry will help tremendously relieve the stress that children can experience when they keep things bottled up inside.

## Validate Your Child

Children need positive environments to flourish. Take the time as parents to observe your child's strengths and comment on their talents and gifts.

Every child has something in which they excel — notice that in your child and comment on it as much as you can. Encourage their talents no matter what they may be. Some children excel in sports, others in math and science, and many excel in the arts. Whatever your child's interests are, be sure to encourage them to explore that interest. This strategy helps to decrease anger and low self-esteem in your child because they are being validated for who they are, and it will keep them from persistently comparing themselves to others in school or within the family. Offer each sibling the same time and encouragement of their own skills and talents so that each child will feel validated for their unique qualities.

## Game Playing

When children play, they learn. This is a well-known quote because it is the truth. Setting aside play time with your child gives them the amount of personal and individual attention they need to feel reassured that they are loved and cherished for who they really are. Playtime allows children to experience the fact that as a parent, you enjoy their company. This assures them that you see them as people that you want to spend time with. It will increase the positive thoughts a child can have about themselves and their own personalities. Depending upon the age of your child, of course, the games will vary. Puzzles are a great choice for most children and teens. Role-playing with dolls and toys are great for toddlers through 8 or 9 years old. For pre-teens and teens, you may want to engage in outdoor activities like football games, golf, basketball, walking together, or taking a run. Hiking is also a great choice for children old enough to undertake the task. This game playing can be video games as well. Video games will teach you as a parent what your kids are actually interested in and give you the opportunity to monitor the amount of negativity and violence your child may be experiencing.

## Reverse Role-Playing

Reverse role-playing is another strategy parents can use to help their children with anxiety issues because it allows the two parties to see in each other through the other's eyes. Reverse role-playing can be acted out by the parent asking a question like, "How does Mommy react when you bring home a low grade from school?" The child can then show the parent how they experience the reaction, though the parent may not mean it that way, this is how the child sees it. During reversal role-playing, the parent can act as they see the child, maybe giving incomplete answers to the parent's questions about the grade, and can show the child how this can cause frustration for the parent when they are not clear with their answers. This whole process helps to clear the air of assumptions. The child may otherwise be thinking that the parent is angry about the low grade when you as the parent may just be disappointed because you know they can do better. Reverse role-playing is helpful in relieving childhood anxiety because it will show them how you as a parent really feel and this may not be what they have concocted in their minds.

## Avoid Any Talk That's Negative

Avoid any kind of talk that is even bordering on negativity. In fact, avoid negativity altogether if you can help it. Whenever you notice your child is saying something that reflects negativity, put a stop to it and tell them it is important to focus on what is positive instead. Encourage them and work with them to make an active effort to turn their thoughts around.

## Picking Your Top Qualities

This is an exercise you can work on with your child. Ask them to pick three things about themselves that they like. It can be anything from what they're wearing, what they like, or what their favorite feature is. Depending on how young your child is, they may require some help identifying a favourite three. Once they have picked three qualities that they like, encourage them to repeat how much they like it. Do this every day until they can say it with belief and even with a smile on their face. This helps to reaffirm that there are positive qualities to focus on and that they can draw on this during the moment where they feel anxious and might need a little reassurance.

## Celebrate Their Success

Each time your child successfully accomplished something, make a big show and celebration out of it. It doesn't matter if it's something small or major, what matters is to make the child feel that each accomplishment is something that they should be proud of. To give them a reason to smile. A ray of sunshine amidst the anxiety that they are dealing with. This helps to boost their self-worth and let them know repeatedly how proud you are of them. Even more so if that achievement is bringing them one step closer out of their anxiety. It helps to remind them to feel good about themselves again, which is something that they desperately need.

## Use Positive Affirmations with Your Child

Positive affirmations are not just for adults. Children can greatly benefit from them too. Positive affirmations can do remarkable wonders to help shift your child's perception, and it could be just what they need to help them overcome their anxiety. Not only does it help to boost their self-esteem, but it encourages them to feel good about themselves once more. Give your child some options of positive affirmations and ask them to choose one or two that they like best.

Recite them with your child like a daily mantra, do it together with them over and over again. Affirmations help remind your child that they are good enough just the way that they are, and that they are loveable, wonderful, and special.

**Give Your Child Compliments**

Anxiety can be a very thing to process for a child, and they need all the positivity and goodness that they can get. Shower your child with compliments each time you get a chance to, never miss a single opportunity. Put a smile on your child's face and compliment them each day, even if it is something as simple as, "*Your dress looks lovely today*" or "*I love the way you always greet me each morning.*" Just like positive affirmations, this will help motivate and encourage your child's self-esteem, to give them the boost that they need and to shift their focus away from the anxiety that they are feeling. Shower your child with love and compassion and advise them with the best of intentions. Go out of your way to show them they always have your support no matter what, whether they have good days or bad. Simply by using the right words, you can make a huge difference in your child's mood and the way that they feel.

These strategies are simplistic enough that you don't need a degree in psychology to perform. It is important to instill confidence and self-esteem in your child from a young age if you want those teachings to stick with them in the long run. It is harder to work with children in their teens but certainly not impossible. You can still use these strategies to get to know your child better and to get to know when something is going wrong within their worlds. It is important for parents to be positive role models, handling their own problems and issues in a positive manner creating true solutions to their own problematic situations so that they can be role models for their children in this manner. When children see true communication and real problem solving within the home, they will take on those traits and learn to handle their own problems through communication and inquiry.

## Help Your Child Identify Triggers

A big part of helping your child to manage their anxiety includes teaching them and raising awareness about what anxiety is. It also helps to teach them the triggers that could be causing their anxiety and help them identify it, so it doesn't seem too scary. To a child, the unknown can be something that is terrifying, and the more you can help them understand what is happening to them, the better they will learn to cope. Spend some time teaching your child about anxiety awareness and how the triggers are potentially affecting their behaviours and their emotions. Helping them understand the source of their fear shows them that this is something which can be managed and that they have nothing to worry about. Sometimes the triggers could be clear, sometimes they are not, so you would have to spend some time identifying together with your child what their potential trigger causes could be.

For example, if you know social settings causes your child anxiety, you could come up with some coping methods to work on together with your child. Teach them how to cope with the situation rather than run away from it, because social settings are unavoidable.

## Encourage Your Child to Be Healthy

A healthy body and mind is one that is better able to cope with change and adversity. It is important that you encourage your child to always look after themselves, and that health is an important part of life they should never neglect. Encourage your child to exercise and play as much as possible. Physical activity is good for their wellbeing and development. Eating the right foods is also important in staying strong and healthy. Opt for food choices which are high in omega 3, probiotics, fruits, nuts, and yogurt are great for keeping anxiety at bay. You should also ensure that your child gets enough rest and sleep each night, as lack of sleep could also potentially be an anxiety trigger.

# Chapter 3: Parenting an Anxious Child

As a parent, how you behave within the family home becomes a mirror for your child's behavior. When parenting an anxious child, one must be mindful of how problems within the home are handled and make it their promise to be an active and positive role model within your child's life. What a child sees is far more important than what you tell them if the two contradict each other. You cannot say to a child, "Always talk about your worries" if you never speak honestly about your own. Your parental behavior must reflect what you teach your child or it will only confuse them and leave them void of what to do when they are feeling anxiety symptoms.

An anxious child must be taught that life will come with its issues and problems, but that there are calm ways in which they all can be handled. It does not help an anxious child to be told that the world is a fairytale but what does help is that as a parent, you teach real solutions to real problems. The child will then learn that when they have an issue or a stressful situation, there is a solution that will assist in handling that issue. They will not feel so overwhelmed by everyday troubles but instead participate in the strategies they were taught in the earlier chapter.

Anxiety symptoms are temporary though distressing, but it is vital that a child is taught that the symptoms will pass. Do not try to negate or eliminate the feeling your child is experiencing but instead soothe them by letting them know that there is a meaningful solution to the problem. Teach them that though they may feel bad right now, time will assist in relieving that feeling and work together with your child to solve the problem. Allow them to speak it out loud and sit with that emotion knowing that it will pass soon enough.

Don't teach your child the avoidance way of life. Teaching them to avoid stressful situations will only help in the short run and make their anxiety even more intense in the long run because they never learned to truly deal with a problem. Remember that you cannot protect them from every problem in life. This is impossible. However, you can teach them to deal with the temporary anxious feeling while helping to provide solutions.

Remain positive while your child is going through their anxiety symptoms. You can still be realistic with your child about the situation. If your child is stressing over turning a low grade around in a week, explain to your child that a week may not be enough time realistically but if he or she sets their mind to it, they can raise their grades in a semester. This offers a positive solution to a stressful situation. Stay positive without being unrealistic.

Allow your child to feel what they are feeling and give respect to those feelings. You can do this without encouraging negative or sad feelings. Simply listening cannot be a better thing to do when your child is having an episode. This way you can validate their feelings without exacerbating them with your words and judgment. You are enabling them to speak their peace without encouraging them to wallow in those feelings. Focus on solutions always. By focusing on solutions, you can let your child be in the moment, though the moment may be challenging, they will also have a knowing that these problems can be worked out.

Be mindful of your body language and tone of voice when your child is expressing anxiety symptoms. You don't want to make their stress increase by the way you act or sound. Don't increase the severity of their symptoms with negativity. Negativity and truth are two different things. You can be truthful with your child about certain outcomes possible, but don't sound or act worried or stressed out about the situation. What an anxious child needs most are encouragement and reassurance, not doubtful and worrisome feelings added to their own.

Try to be a great model of problem-solving for your child. Remember that you as the parent are your child's most important and effective role model. Sit with your anxious child and work together to create solutions to their problems and worries. Make it a family affair to sit with your child and focus on ideas to help with their issue at hand. The more an anxious child receives support and the teachings of real problem solving, the easier it will be for them to handle anxious feelings that arise, knowing that most situations can be handled with peace and positive thinking.

Teach your child healthy ways of handling their anxiety symptoms. Even young children are now learning meditation techniques and the use of aromatherapy to help calm their nerves. Be an example as a parent by using some of these techniques to handle your own problems and anxiety issues. Most importantly, be honest with your child and allow them to see that everything is not always perfect for you. This will make them feel so much more comfortable telling you about their anxiety and sharing their feelings with you.

As a parent of an anxious child, it is vital that you set the example of how to communicate and handle life's problems.

## 5 Steps to Building a Better Connection with Your Anxious Child

Building a better emotional connection between you and your child begins with you because your child will be unable to properly manage and deal with their emotions, let alone be able to ask for help. Here are 5 steps to building a better connection with your child to help them through this anxious period of their life.

- **Encourage Your Child Not to Be Afraid** - Nobody can be strong all the time, and even the strongest of people sometimes need someone to lean on for support. Even more so for a child, who is only just starting to make sense of the world and process their emotions as they are growing into adulthood. Encourage your child to never be afraid to ask for support and help. Let them know that it is not a sign of weakness, that whenever it feels like something is getting too hard to bear to always seek help. Let them know they can come to you and the two of you will work together to overcome what troubles them. Working through a problem together will bring the two of you closer, and it helps build that bond of trust because you know you can rely on each other when it matters most.

- **Always Be Honest with Your Child** - It is important to be open and honest whenever you communicate with your child. This is how you build and strengthen the bond of trust between you. Even if your first instinct may be to protect and shield them from the truth, think about it for a moment and weigh the pros and cons of being honest with them depending on the situation. Being able to comfortably express yourself and to encourage your child to do the same will help show them that there is nothing to be afraid of.

- **Encourage Your Child to Always Look Forward, Never Back** - The past should remain in the past where it belongs. If your child has been traumatized by a previous experience, reassure them that just because something bad happened in the past, it doesn't mean that it is going to happen all the time. Encourage them to look at it as something which they l        d from, an experience which makes        i stronger. Talk about the past experi if it helps and help them look a experience from a different perspe ...u. Share your own experiences with them, and talk about how you moving forward did a great deal to help you overcome what you were afraid of.

- **Encourage Your Child to Express Gratitude** - Expressing gratitude is a great bonding tool which will bring the two of you closer together. Not only that, but it infuses positive feelings and gives your child something to smile about. Often in times of anxiety, it can be easy to forget about the many things that we all have to be grateful for. The bad times and the worries seem much worse and our minds can't focus on anything else except that. Especially for a child who has not quite reached the emotional maturity needed to compartmentalize their feelings. Encourage your child to engage in gratitude exercises with you. Talk about the things that you are grateful for and encourage them to do the same. Let them know you appreciate them letting you into their world. Let them know you love and appreciate them for who they are. Let them know that you're grateful they put their trust in you, to come and talk to you about their problems.

- **Encourage Your Child with Baby Steps** - You don't have to have a deep heart-to-heart with your child immediately. You could end up overwhelming them and making things worse. Start small with baby steps in the beginning. Talk about one thing at the time and gauge your child's comfort level before you move on.

Taking baby steps will slowly encourage your child to come out of their shell when they see they can trust you enough to unload their problems by talking to you about it. The more they trust you, the more open they will become. It is about forging that bond and gaining their trust because children are at a tender and fragile age. They need a pillar of strength that they can lean on and this is where you play a very important role in their lives.

# Chapter 4: Engaging Games and Crafts for Parents and Children

Game playing can be a great and effective tactic to help your child deal with and manage their anxiety symptoms. Below is a list of games proven to assist you and your child with dealing with many of the anxiety symptoms we have discussed earlier in this book.

### Topple

Topple is a more grown-up version of Don't Spill the Beans. It encourages dexterity and patience and requires a child to follow directions. Most of all, it is fun to play with parents and this in itself will calm a child down when experiencing anxiety symptoms. Topple has different physical levels. You or your child rolls the die and a number pops up. This number tells you where you can place your pawn piece. There are numbers located on the board on each level. This causes your child to focus on something other than the symptoms they may currently be experiencing. Topple is appropriate is for ages 6 and up.

### Pop the Pig

For younger children, ages 4 and up, Pop the Pig is an effective game for helping to decrease childhood anxiety symptoms. Again, in the Pop the Pig, a board game, everyone takes a turn rolling the die which engages the entire family. This is a great game to involve both parents if both parents are living within the home at the time, along with any other siblings the anxiety-ridden child may have.

## Uno Attack

Uno Attack is for ages 7 and up. The most important thing about game playing is that it engages the child and parent in a thinking activity that places the symptoms of anxiety further down on the worry list. As a child plays, they learn and learning utilizes parts of the brain often taken up by worry and stress. Uno Attack is a version of the original Uno card game that is played by two players only. This allows for some special time between the parent and child and parents can take turns engaging with the child in this version of the game. It will make the child feel just how special they are to you. This builds confidence and eases worry symptoms.

## Worry Stones

Since worrying is a huge part of childhood anxiety symptoms, making these worry stones can be done together with one or both parents. At your local craft store, buy oven clay that can be baked. While shopping, ask your child to choose 3 colors that appeal to them. The child will make balls out of this clay and imprint the balls with fingerprints, peaceful words or mantras, anything that makes the child feel happy and calm. The stones get baked in the oven and the child can carry them to school, camp, or to any social activity that may trigger anxiety. These stones are often called "Reminder" stones because they remind the child to think of fun, loving, and calm thoughts when they may be away from you, their support system.

**Mantra Jewelry**

Mantra Jewelry can be made in a few ways. You can go to your favorite craft store and get bracelet making kits with paper included so that you and your child can write positive mantras on the jewelry. Words like, "I have support", "I am loved", or "I am strong", are just a few of the mantras that you and your child can include in this project. This activity, along with the Worry Stones is perfect for when your child is away from home. They both act as reminders of their support system at home.

**Make a Journal**

Get together with your child and help them create a journal. Something handwritten in which they can work out their issues and feelings. A journal will create the opportunity for you and your child to speak about how they are feeling, a chance to discuss their worries and fear. A journal will also create a way for your child to look back and see how far they have come by handling their anxiety symptoms in a healthy and creative way.

## Make a Worry-Free Toolbox

Take all your child's crafts and games and put them in a big toy box or chest. This will make a worry-free toolbox for them to visit during their anxiety crisis. They can go to this toolbox and pull out a favorite game to play or a piece of mantra jewelry that will remind them that everything will be alright in time. The toolbox will be their refuge for handling anxiety symptoms as they arise, and you can go through the toolbox with your child and decide what they may need the most, a game or a craft reminder. This is another way you can be engaged with your child when they are dealing with anxiety issues.

## I've Got Butterflies in My Tummy

This is a wonderful activity which will get your child to open up and give you the perfect opportunity to talk to them about what worries them or even what they're afraid of. All you need to do to get started is to cut out templates of butterflies in different sizes. Next, trace an outline of your child on another piece of paper and cut that out. Now, talk to your child about all the physical sensations they are likely to experience within their body whenever they feel worried or scared. For example, how it feels to have "butterflies in your tummy". You can end each session with calming, breathing exercises and giving your child a hug — a comforting hug at the end of it. Put the butterflies in a net that you've drawn or cut out and show them that you'll always be there to help them catch the butterflies when they need you.

## Using Stress Balls

This is one even adults rely on to help them calm their nerves in times of stress and it is great for kids because of the sensory element involved. Your child will love holding, rolling, and squeezing the ball between their hands. If you don't have a stress ball, no problem — it is very easy to make one of your own. Simply fill a balloon with either flour, rice, or even play dough. Don't forget to double wrap the balloon at the end to ensure that it is nice and secure. We don't want any of that stuff falling out. Each time your child is nervous and anxious, distract them by using the stress ball. Shifting their focus away from their anxiety with an enjoyable activity will help them forget what is making them so nervous in the first place.

## My Little Calming Jar

This is another great one that kids will love. Calming jars can be a source of "security" for your child and it is very easy to make too. All you need is a jar, fill it with some warm water, and add glitter glue into the mix. You're done! Plastic jars would be best, in this case, to ensure that there's no breakage or risk of an injury happening. All your child needs to do is shake it each time they feel nervous or anxious. It is a fantastic tool which helps them calm down because there is just something about watching all that glitter float around that has a calming element to it. They can keep it in their room with them, or if they want to bring it with them on the go, you can easily recreate this in smaller, travel sized plastic bottles. Easy peasy!

**I'm A Superhero**

Get your little ones especially to imagine their favorite superhero. You could either get them the costumes or make them yourself to really get into the role-playing. Encourage your child to imagine that they are superheroes too and that they are fighting off the "bad guys" (their anxieties and worries) because they are strong, brave, and capable of doing anything they set their mind to. This is a great way to indirectly encourage and remind your kids that there's nothing to be afraid of, that they are strong enough to do anything. All they have to do is pretend to be a superhero or think what their favorite superhero would do if they were afraid. Ask your child what powers they wished they had and what they would use them for (this will give you a lot of insight into your child's innermost fears and what they wished they could do to make it go away). You could even encourage them to draw their favorite superhero fighting off the bad guy. There are a lot of possibilities with this activity.

**A Walk with Nature**

Instead of being cooped up at home, get your anxious child moving by taking them for a walk to change up the environment. Exercise is a great way to improve their mood, and there's nothing like a change of scenery to take their mind of what's worrying them. It removes your child from the anxiety triggers while at the same time giving them exercise and a chance to breathe in all that fresh air. You could also take this time to point out all the beauty that nature has to offer. This could help them calm down significantly and feel much happier in the process. It is also a great way to bond with your child as you take them to their favorite spots and point out all the beautiful things that the two of you see along the way.

**Just Dance!**

Rhythm and movement are something that every child love. Kids love to sing and dance to their favorite tunes because it makes them happy and brings them great joy. This is why there could be no better tool to fall back on then just dancing!

Whenever your child is feeling anxious, get their favorite tunes out and encourage them to get up and dance. Do it along with them! The little ones especially love this, and it is such an engaging activity which can immediately lift their spirits and make them forget what it was they were so anxious about before. Music is capable of bringing so much joy and comfort. It is no wonder children love it. Create a playlist of all the songs that you notice your kids love to sing and dance to and have them on standby. When the time comes, all you need to do is hit play and just dance along with them. Let your inner child loose and just have fun as you bond with your child.

## Apps That Help Your Kids with Anxiety

The beauty of living in the digital age is that we've got all sorts of tools at our disposal to help with just about any kind of situation including how to parent a child with anxiety. Aside from games and engaging craft projects which you could work on with them, another great tool is to make use of the available apps out there designed to help anxious kids just like yours.

Here are some of the apps you might find useful.

### The Positive Penguins App

Originally created by an 11-year old Australian child and her two brothers, this app helps your child learn and understand positive ways of interpreting situations. This app is designed to help kids sort through what they are feeling. It helps children understand and identify how their feelings are influenced by their thoughts. It helps the child take the thoughts which were ambiguous and intangible before and make them easy to understand. The app provides a platform for your child to either speak about what they're feeling or to type it out. There is also a forum to be found within the app which identifies negative thoughts and helps the child learn how to identify them. This app is suitable for children aged 9 to 11 years old.

**The Bedtime Meditations for Kids App**

This is a great app for helping kids drift off into a sleep which is calm and peaceful. When your child is anxious and worried, their minds never seem to quiet down, even when they are about to go to bed. For the child with an overactive mind, Bedtime Meditations for Kids helps your child take their mind off of their anxieties and focus on calming thoughts, which will help them settle down so they can peacefully fall asleep and get the much-needed rest they deserve after a long day. This app is suitable for children up to the age of 12 years-old.

**The Breathe2Relax App**

This app was designed to be used as a stress reduction tool for kids. Anxiety makes your child's breathing become shallow and ragged, which only serves to ramp up their anxiety levels even more. For those moments when you need to help your child calm down but you don't have anything on hand to help you with the situation, Breathe2Relax is a good app to fall back on. Think of it as your portable stress management tool for your child. It helps them use deep breathing as a way to calm their nerves, and over time as they get accustomed to these exercises, it will help them better manage and cope with their anxieties, especially when they're not at home. This app is suitable for children ages 6+.

**The Songza App**

Can you think of anything more calming than relaxing music? The old saying *"music doth soothe the savage beast"* says a lot about the powerful impact that music can have on the human brain. For an anxious child, nothing could be a more wonderful tool than having music to calm them down. Songza is a wonderful app that streams music which is helpful in calming your child down. It allows your child to choose the music option based on the activity or the time of day, depending on their preference. This app is suitable for children aged 13+.

Engaging with your child is vital to understanding what triggers their anxiety worries and is highly important to help them decrease the symptoms. Whether playing a board game to help them focus their minds on something fun or using crafts to create positive reminders, spending time with your child that is private and personal is a highly effective way to assist your child in expressing their emotions when suffering from anxiety disorder.

# Chapter 5: Depression vs. Anger

Life is challenging enough without having to deal with depression, especially for a child. Depression can make everyday life a struggle for anyone who is experiencing it, and in the eyes of a child, on top of everything else they have to deal with, it can seem almost impossible to find happiness with this black cloud in your life.

There are several differences between depression and anger, although both can be triggered by the same circumstance. In this chapter, we will explain the differences first and then how you can deal with both these emotions when it comes to your child's anxiety worries.

**Depression**

Sadness is a normal emotion for all of us. It is a low or down feeling that is usually caused by a specific circumstance or event such as loss of a loved one, someone we love being hurt or injured, or any form of disappointment or grief. This is not the same condition as depression. Depression can be described as sadness taken to a deeper level. It is a constant sadness or a void of all feelings. The child may not feel anything whatsoever and may be incapable of even feeling sad. True depression is a form of sadness that lingers and can be debilitating and interfere with your child's normal activities.

Depression is the black hole of feelings whereas normal sadness is a temporary occurrence. When your child is depressed, the condition may last for weeks, even months, and it appears to them that there is no way out of these dark feelings. Dealing with depression is different than dealing with normal sadness or anger, which we will discuss later in this chapter. True depression can also be a sign that something is biologically unbalanced. With depression, a visit to a doctor may be required to locate the underlying cause.

Often parents can be at a loss when it comes to dealing with their child's depression. However, there are effective ways to help your child should they be going this particular mood disorder. Once it has been determined that there is no biological cause for your child's depression, there are a few ways in which to handle this debilitating condition.

For a child, depression can make life feel seem unbearable and like a constant struggle. The feelings of despair, hopelessness, and unhappiness that cannot be explained could threaten to down them in what seems like a never-ending cycle of misery. If left untreated, this can even spiral into suicidal thoughts and tendencies, which is already venturing into dangerous territory. If you suspect that your child may be dealing with depression, don't ignore the signs and brush it off as something that will eventually pass.

**Anger**

Anger, on the other hand, can often be mistaken for depression because it feels almost the same. Almost, but not quite. Admittedly, it can sometimes be hard to distinguish one from the other, especially for a child. This is why it often falls on the parents to try and help them make the distinction.

Anger can often be an emotion which fuels depression, but it is most certainly different. Anger is described as an emotional and physiological result or response towards a situation. It often rears its head when a perceived threat is present. In more severe instances, anger can often lead to aggressive behavior patterns.

You will usually be able to clearly identify anger as it is often accompanied by angry expressions, shouting, arguments and it is often not subtle. Far from it sometimes, depending on how angry your child may be feeling. Anger can often manifest itself physically in both adults and child. You can feel your blood pressure start to rise, your facial expression changes, sometimes you even ball your hands into fists, clenching them hard just to control your emotions. A child may display these same signs which are what you want to look out for.

Anger often makes an appearance as a direct result of an action or situation. This emotion can be just as bad as depression is, because it can create and trap your child in an ugly cycle which can be hard to escape from. A young child may not know how to properly express their emotions, often using phrases like "*I hate you*" or "*everything sucks!*" to convey their feelings of anger.

## What You Can Help Your Child Do to Overcome Depression

If your child is in fact, dealing with depression, there is something that can help — Meditation. In fact, this method can be used even if your child is dealing with anger. Meditation is a good remedy for both. Meditation has been the practice that has been used for centuries to achieve mental well-being and happiness, satisfaction, and emotional stability. It is not just something that is for adults, anyone at any age can begin adopting this practice. In fact, why not practice it with the whole family. Get everyone involved so your child feels the added security of having familial support on their side.

Meditation helps you find yourself and connect your mind with your body so you once more feel like you are in control of everything that is happening to you. It works because it minimizes and reduces the risk of experiencing depression by helping to put a stop to the production of excess cortisol in your child's body. Cortisol has been known to cause many stress-related disorders which include depression. Meditation is also effective in helping to balance the neurotransmitters in the brain, especially dopamine and serotonin which have been strongly linked to causing depression.

Meditation will also be a useful exercise if your child is experiencing anger issues. This is because it teaches your child to focus on controlling their mind, to that they can eventually learn to control the negative chatter and thoughts which may be running around in their head, robbing them of their happiness. It teaches your child how to control their breathing, increasing the blood circulation in their brain to deliver the essential nutrients, energy, and oxygen that it needs to function properly. For a growing child, this is important because a healthy brain is much better at fighting off depression.

Helping your child overcome depression is going to be an uphill battle and possibly a long road to recovery. You need to do everything that you can to help your child along the process and ensure they are fully reaping the benefits of the meditative experience. That means helping your child find the right type of meditation that is going to be the most comfortable to help them deal with the process. If this is the first time both you and your child are attempting meditation, there is the option of guided meditation to make the process much easier. In fact, it is recommended that children try guided meditation to begin easing into the practice because the verbal cues and aid can help provide them with the support that they need to ensure they are on the right track.

## How Meditation Will Be Beneficial in Helping Your Child Overcome Anger and Depression

Your child stands to gain a lot by using meditation to help them overcome their depression and anger issues. The great thing about meditation is how easily this tool is accessible to anyone who wants to harness its benefits in the fight against depression. Meditation is so beneficial because it works on improving the soul, body, and the mind, which makes achieving overall health and wellness entirely possible. It is easy to follow, which makes it suitable for any age group. With a child, you will want to practice along with them, to guide them along the way and ensure they're on the right track.

Overcoming depression is no easy feat and your child is going to require a lot of support along the way. In the beginning, meditation might be a struggle for your child, especially when it comes to trying to maintain their focus and not be easily distracted having their thoughts wander back to what is making them miserable. Over time, with repetitive practice, meditation will help to enhance your child's focus and concentration, and by sticking to this practice, they will eventually learn to gain control over their thoughts and improve their mindfulness.

Children, especially teenagers, are at a very crucial point in their life. They are learning to reshape their thoughts as they learn to adapt to new experiences. It is important that as parents, you are there to help them develop a positive view of the world so that they will grow up to become well-rounded adults who will go out into the world and be the successful people you know they can be.

Some of the benefits that your child stands to gain by adopting meditation as a way of dealing with their anger and depression include the following:

- A reduction in their stress levels.

- Improved sleep quality, which is very important for children who are still in the growing phase of their life.

- Helps to boost feelings of peace, calm, serenity, and happiness.

- Makes negative situations seem more manageable and less overwhelming.

- It supports healthy emotional development.

## Easy Ways Your Child Can Learn to Meditate

Meditation is something that requires patience, discipline, time, and commitment, which are also crucial skills your child should be learning to develop as they grow into young adults. For your child to experience the full benefits of meditation, you must help them establish a firm practice which takes place every day if possible and maintain meditation with consistency.

- **Help Your Child Choose a Place** - Set up a quiet spot in your home where your child (and you) can meditate in a calm setting. Find a comfortable area in your home where you and your child can obtain complete privacy and quiet. Understandably, this might be tricky if there are siblings or other family members present, but what you could do is talk to them and let them know what you're doing.

- **Help them with the Right Positions and Postures** - Meditation is something that is going to require your child to do a lot of breathing. For this purpose, you need to help them work on getting your posture exactly right during your meditational sessions so that they can breathe deeply and meaningfully the way it is intended.

- **Help Them Set a Time** - Help your child come to see meditation as a regular part of their everyday routine. Make it a habit to devote a certain period of time purely just for your meditational sessions, much like you would with other routines you're used to doing. Help them ease into the process by starting small at first, even doing it together with them. As a start, try 5 or 10-minute segment blocks which are easily accomplished and doable. Then move onto increasing those time blocks in stages until your child can comfortably meditate without getting easily distracted.

## Reassure Your Child to Never Give Up

Everything can seem hopeless when your child feels nothing but despair. As a parent, one of the best things you can do for them is to reassure them to never give up, especially on their dreams. Overcoming depression is a long process which involves continuous effort. If your child is a teenager, let them know that they should never give up working towards their dreams because depression and anger is something they can overcome.

Motivated them to keep working on their dreams by:

- **Encouraging them to Set Smaller Goals** - Smaller goals are more attainable. When your child is depressed, their dreams may seem almost impossible to achieve because they feel so unhappy. Help them set smaller, more attainable goals first and help them work towards achieving those targets. Each small goal they accomplish is a small victory that gives them an extra boost of happiness and reminds them that each goal achieved is bringing them one step closer to the bigger dream they have in mind.

- **Help Them Take It One Day at a Time** - Don't try to do too much too soon. Give yourself and your child time to take a break and remember that some things take time. Take it one day at a time, and remember, if you don't succeed today, there is always tomorrow.

- **Encourage them to Write It Down** - Writing things down and sticking it where we can see it in front of our eyes every day is a great way to keep reminding ourselves of what could otherwise be so easily forgotten. It works the same way for adults and for kids. Sometimes your child needs a reminder that no matter what circumstances they may be going through, it is important to never give up on what they love and what they want. Remind your child constantly that every day is a brand-new day, situations change, and five or ten years from now, they could find themselves in a completely different place from where they are today. Remind them to never give up on their dreams, keep chasing them because they never know where it will lead them to in life.

# Chapter 6: Panic Attacks vs Fear

## The Difference between Panic Attacks and Fear

Fear and panic attacks are both conditions which could overlap and sometimes they could be mistaken and interchanged with one another. However, in no way they are the same. Despite the fact that both these traits produce a stress response, fear is most certainly a very different emotion from that of panic attacks.

The difference between fear and panic attacks is that the former is caused by a known threat, something that is easily understood. Like a fear of spiders for example. Panic attacks, on the other hand, is part of a symptom which often accompanies anxiety. Fear induces within all of us — not just children — our primal fight or flight response, something which comes out in moments where we feel "threatened". Our ancestors used it to survive in the wild and the human species has survived for as long as it did because of this fight or flight reaction.

Both children and adults experience fear when there is a defined threat present. An example of a child's fear would be a fear of the dark or the fear of being alone in a room by themselves at night. A fear of spiders maybe. This type of "danger" is something that can easily be defined and understood. There is a clear focus about what it is they are afraid of. That is the definition of fear.

Panic attacks, on the other hand, are something entirely different. The best way to describe it would be a fear that is magnified to a whole new level.

Panic attacks and anxiety too are often thought to be interchangeable, and while they do share some similarities, there are slight differences between the two. Panic attacks are a common occurrence when a person is suffering from anxiety, and if your child is showing signs of this, this could be what they are dealing with.

Panic attacks often occur when a person is experiencing high levels of stress or worrying excessively. Some of the common symptoms of a panic attack include increase breathing pace, an increase in the heart rate, difficulty breathing, shortness of breath, sweating profusely, and even dizziness for some. A child may also experience these same symptoms as they are not exclusively for adults alone. A panic attack is different from that of regular fear because this is fear on an intensified level. Sometimes, it is not even fear anymore but extreme terror, apprehension for some people and for others, and sheer nervousness. With panic attacks, the symptoms can be so extreme that they often cause a disruption in the daily routine. If your child is experiencing a panic attack, you will find that they are suddenly unable to function, they lose all sense of self, and they won't be able to function normally let alone follow simple, basic instructions. They need excessive amounts of comforting to help them to calm down.

The length of a panic attack would differ based on the individual. Some attacks may last longer than others, although they eventually do subside after a while. It is difficult to predict when a panic attack may strike. If you suspect that your child may be suffering from panic attacks, keep an eye out for symptoms which include excessive sweating, visible trembling, shaking, unsteadiness on their feet, pounding heartbeats, and irrational fear like they are losing control, maybe even some hysterical behavior.

## What Is Anxiety and Panic Attacks?

It is common for everyone to feel worried from time to time. Have you ever known anyone who has lived a completely worry-free life? No, because it is not possible. We all experience worry at some point in our lives because those types of emotions are both natural and unavoidable. It is not just adults who can experience anxiety, but children too.

Experiencing a little bit of anxiety and sadness throughout the different stages of life is completely normal. When does it stop being normal? When it begins to feel like fear and worries are the emotions that seem to dominate the bigger part of your day, every day.

## Does Your Child Have Anxiety?

Anxiety can often cause panic attacks and great distress, especially for a child. Although it is normal for everyone to worry from time to time, excessive worry and distress can often lead to panic attacks and anxiety. When does normal worry stop being normal and cross over into anxiety? Well, there is a fine line between both. To tell if your child is suffering from anxiety, the following symptoms will help you identify it:

- **Your Child Feels Crippled By Their Fears** - Being afraid of something is one thing, being so crippled by that fear that they become unable to think or react rationally – or sometimes not being able to react at all – is another tell-tale sign of anxiety disorder.

- **Your Child Has Difficulty Sleeping** - Does your child find themselves lying awake in bed at night, worried, stressed, agitated, or nervous? No matter how much you try to coax them to sleep, it simply isn't working? Insomnia or trouble falling asleep because of worry is a sure sign that what your child may be dealing with is anxiety or panic attacks.

- **Your Child Has Trouble Focusing** - Anxious thoughts will have a way of consuming your child without them even noticing that they're slowly taking over. Difficulty concentrating on even the simplest of tasks because their mind either goes blank or starts to worry again is another sign that your child could be dealing with anxiety.

- **They Find It Difficult to Let Go** - To someone dealing with anxiety, letting go is not easy. Even more so for a child. When your child is dealing with anxiety, they will be prone to overthinking situations, sometimes reliving traumatic and negative moments from their past experience. They have a hard time forgetting and letting go of past hurt and pain, which can cause them a great deal of suffering when they don't quite know how to deal with it appropriately.

- **Frequent Panic Attack Episodes** - If your child is experiencing a sense of helplessness and gripped by fear that starts to manifest itself physically in the form of a panic attack, your child could be dealing with anxiety. Common symptoms include sweat, feeling weak, dizzy, experience chest and stomach pains, feel nauseous, and have difficulty breathing, what you've got on your hands is most definitely an anxiety disorder.

- **Your Child Is Tense and Agitated All the Time** - Anxiety will leave your child feeling tense and stressed and a side effect of that which is going to manifest itself physically is muscle aches and soreness.

- **They Seem to Get Tired Easily** - Anxiety is a very draining emotion and no one can truly understand how much it can impact a person unless they themselves are dealing with anxiety.

- **Their Panic Attacks Get Triggered by Change** - Whether you have anxiety or not, having a comfort zone which you do not want to leave is a very normal occurrence. If you sometimes find it hard to cope with change as an adult, imagine how much harder it is for a child? Even for a normal person, sometimes taking a step out of the comfort zone can prove to be a challenge, so for a person — a child no less — who is dealing with anxiety, those feelings are much worse. They are resistant to change because they fear the unknown and they are terrified that their worst fears will come true so they find it difficult to accept change. Your child is going to require a lot of support to cope with this, and you need to be patient with them.

## Why Is My Child Experiencing Panic Attacks and Anxiety?

It could be a combination of one or several factors. It is difficult to identify what specifically causes anxiety because different people have different triggers and don't always respond necessarily in the same way. Anxiety could stem from genetics if some people in your family have had to deal with this condition before. Anxiety is a condition with a genetic predisposition and if your family has had a history of dealing with anxiety, that's probably why your child is currently experiencing the same thing.

Anxiety very much depends on the individual and it is affected by certain traits like their personality, current health, lifestyle, and the things that have happened to them in the past. Your child could also potentially develop anxiety if they are constantly exposed to ongoing stressful situations. Stressful events here could be anything from stress at school, a change in your living environment, an emotional episode which has caused them great emotional distress, and even the social situations they may have to deal with.

Because it could be caused by several potential elements, anxiety and panic attacks are tricky symptoms to pinpoint. Anxiety can manifest itself in different aspects of a person's life, which is why even children are able to experience anxiety, although they may not fully understand what is happening to them.

## Understanding Anxiety

By now, it is pretty clear that anxiety and fear are two very different things. Fear will not cause your child to break out into panic attacks. Anxiety will. To better understand what your child may be going through, it is important for the parents to know a couple of key facts about anxiety which will put you in a better position to offer your child the support that they need during this difficult time.

- Anxiety is a very real problem that is not to be taken lightly.

- Anxiety is a serious issue that requires serious help.

- Anxiety is a condition which is normal.

- Anxiety is a mental health issue that should never be dismissed with statements such as its "all in your head".

- Anxiety makes your child a prisoner of their own fears.

- Anxiety makes it hard for your child to live a normal life, even the smallest tasks seem hard to do.

- Anxiety can be a debilitating and crippling disorder because it can prevent your child from functioning normally in an everyday routine.

- Anxiety is not in any way a sign of weakness.

- Anxiety is not something your child can just "get over" as the genuine worries and fear experienced need to be properly dealt with.

## What Is It Like For Your Child to Live With Anxiety?

Anxiety is a human emotion, which means just like all the other emotions we experience as human beings, it is going to vary in intensity depending on the individual. In the case of a child, it can be quite a stressful experience for them especially when they do not fully understand what it is they are going through and why they are feeling this way. Living with anxiety for them can be difficult because they don't know how to effectively express all the emotions that they are feeling. As a result, they may suffer from low self-esteem and find it very difficult to socialize.

When experienced on a severe level, anxiety and panic attack episodes could cause your child to become needy and clingy, always needing reassurance otherwise they would feel lost and insecure. They can become emotionally unstable, swinging from one extreme emotion to another. One minute they could be extremely happy, the next extremely sad or angry for no rhyme or reason. They constantly need to be assured on a daily basis to make them feel better.

They become prone to panic attacks because they feel overwhelmed by their negative emotions. They suffer from insomnia because their mind never seems to stop worrying. It can put a lot of pressure and stress on the relationships that they have because not many people would realize what they're going through and think that they are just overreacting.

## How to Help Your Child Deal and Cope with Anxiety

To help your child cope with the panic attacks they could be struggling with as a result of anxiety, here are some things that you could do.

**Help Your Child Deal with Their Fears**
When your child is suffering from anxiety, there are two primary emotions which they are going to constantly feel — worry and fear which causes the panic attacks. When they are in this state, they find it difficult to trust and connect with anyone including their parents. To help them through it, approach the situation calmly so that you can help to calm them down. Do not react equally emotionally because that could just escalate the situation when they are already in a highly emotional state of mind. You need to remain calm and steady before attempting to calm your child down. A great approach here would be to encourage them to talk to you about what they are feeling. If they don't want to share, don't push them. Give them their space but keep reminding them you are there if they need to talk. This can be a wonderful show of emotional support, something that they desperately need when they're facing a panic attack episode.

**Help Your Child Express Their Emotions**
Children may have trouble expressing how they really feel. They may try to suppress their emotions because they don't know what else to do about it. The more that they try to reject and suppress their emotions, the worse their anxiety may become and it could even end up spiraling

out of control, resulting in a panic attack. You can help the situation by approaching your child with empathy, kindness, and love. Remind them that you are not going anywhere, and if they need someone to talk to, encourage them to trust you enough to open up. This may take some time and much persuasion, though, so you are going to need to exercise a fair amount of patience here to help them through the process. Never stop showering them with love, and never show your impatience because that will only distress them even more than ever.

## Help Your Child by Communicating With Them

Sometimes your child may need a shoulder to cry on, to feel like there is someone who understands them. When you communicate with your child in this situation to help them feel better, you need to use the right words with them. Using the right words can make a huge difference in the direction and outcome of a conversation. For example, use words that reassure them of your love and support, that lets them know without a doubt that you are there for them no matter what. Ask them how they are doing every day, tell them you love them. Everyone likes being told that they are loved and appreciated, even more so if they are suffering from anxiety. It can be difficult to remain positive when things are difficult and challenging, so what you can do to help is to keep reminding your child at every opportunity that they are never alone no matter what they may think.

# Conclusion

Thank you for making it through to the end of this book, let's hope it was informative and able to provide you with all of the tools you need to achieve your goals whatever they may be.

The next step is to use these tools that you've just read about as a building block towards helping your child deal with their anxiety problems, to show them that it is possible to make things better. It is important to let your child know that they are not alone in this journey and you will be there for them every step of the way, in any way that they need.

Your child may be dealing with anxiety, but it is not the end of the world. There is something that can be done to make the situation better, and thanks to this guidebook, you now have all the tools that you need to help your child overcome worry, stress, anger, depression, panic attacks, and fear. This workbook is yours and your child's guide to personal freedom once more.

Helping your child overcome their anxiety is going to be a process which takes time and practice so do not get frustrated if you don't see immediate results. You will eventually get there and more importantly, patience is one of the most vital qualities to have as you work together with your child to overcome this difficult stage.

The tools and information that you will have in this book could mean the difference between your child living a life of loneliness and frustration, being plagued with anxiety, or living a life where they are free, happy, and living it to the fullest being surrounded by friends, family, and even strangers without worrying and being anxious every minute of the day.

Finally, if you found this book useful in any way, a review on Amazon is always appreciated!

Made in the USA
Middletown, DE
03 January 2021

30551951R10044